Activate your Home or Office

For Success in

Health

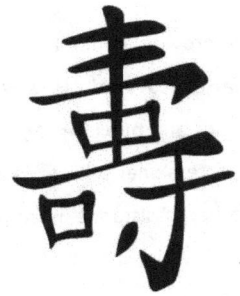

With Feng Shui

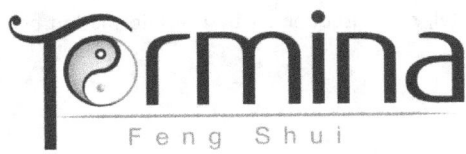

Copyright © 2016 Termina Feng Shui. All rights reserved. No part of this book may be reproduced or transmitted in any form without written permission from the authors and publisher, except for brief inclusion of quotations or for review purposes.First Edition

This book is designed to provide competent and reliable information regarding the subject matter covered. However, it is sold with the understanding that the author and publisher are not engaged in rendering legal, financial, or other professional advice. Laws vary from country to country and if legal or other assistance is required, the services of a professional should be sought. The intent of the author is only to offer information of a general nature to help you in your quest for well-being, the author and the publisher assume no responsibility for your actions. The author shall have no liability or responsibility to any person or entity regarding physical, psychological, emotional, financial, commercial damages, special, incidental, or consequential by the information contained in this book.

Contents

Introduction
What is Feng Shui
Invite your desired health in
Clutter management
Activate your wellness
- General Health
- The Centre
- Quality of air
- Natural light
- Clear space
- Set your Intention

Areas in the environment
- Lounge and Family Room
- Dining Room
- Bedroom
- Bathroom and Kitchen
- Front Door
- Workspace
- Outside Areas
- Body/Home Connection
- Body/Elements
- Geopathic Stress
- Cleansing
- Express Happiness
- General

Health enhancers
- Clarity
- Celebration
- The Trinity of Luck
- Honesty and Honour

- Purity
- Joy
- Transparency
- Faith
- Transformation
- Tenderness
- Balance and Harmony
- Focus
- Compassion
- Empowerment/Self-Empowerment
- Enhance Your Connection to Heaven
- Your Senses

Quick tips

Create a vision Board

Introduction

The importance of wellness is imperative and one that requires to be at the top of our things to achieve. Without good health many areas in our life do not function well, nor can we achieve our fullest potential. If you have problems with any aspects of your health, feel overwhelmed, stressed and lacking in vitality this is the area to concentrate on. Or you may want to maintain the wellness and youthfulness already experienced in your life. Whatever your desire is, create good health for your loved ones and YOU. Feng Shui principles work in harmony with the direct relationship between your health, the quality of energy in your home or workplace and opens the flow of Qi for the health you desire in your life.

The important thing to remember is that your environment is your physical visualisation board and this unconsciously creates your outcomes, 24 hours a day, 7 days a week. The Chinese and now quantum physics teach us that we are surrounded by energy, in fact, everything is energy. Our environment is energy. Einstein told us this *"Everything is energy and that's all there is to it. Match the frequency of the reality you want and you cannot help but get that reality. It can be no other way. This is not philosophy. This is physics."* Energy or energy forces in Feng Shui are termed as Qi (chi). A good flow energy, also known as frequency, leads to abundance, prosperity and happiness while negative energy leads to misfortune and unhappiness.

Whether you are Building, Designing, Buying, Renting, Selling, Living or Working in a premises, Feng Shui improves your life in so many ways. If there is something going on in your life that you wish to change or improve: Health, career, relationships, financial issues, support, business, wealth, or academic achievement. — You name it — it's all possible by adjusting your environment. All of life circumstances fall under the Feng Shui umbrella of possibilities and there is no limit to what you can improve or amplify positively when these ancient principles and science is applied.

With Feng Shui we can arrange our environment so that we receive maximum support with solutions for improvement, maximising the energy of the home or office for the occupants so that there is improvement in the health, wealth and relationship areas of their lives. The 4000 year old art and science of Feng Shui helps harness the power of good energy in the home and cures the effects of negative energy. Many home and business owners confirm to the fact that Feng Shui has helped them with their struggles and even result in a more attractive living or work space.

What is Feng Shui

Feng Shui is a science and ancient art based on laws that govern the flow of energy. The term Feng Shui translates to "wind-water" in English and is a Chinese Metaphysic Art, practised through formulas and calculations using energy forces referred to as Qi (chi). Both Feng and Shui are associated with good health and prosperity which is why the art is so highly regarded in the east. Energy in the environment remains stuck, people are prevented from moving forward, or experience unwanted circumstances, however, by increasing the flow of energy this clears the path to propel forward and to bring to fruition desired intentions. By creating Positive changes in the environment it produces improvements in the level and flow of Qi energy bringing high levels of good fortune and creating a more favourable and harmonious layout for a home or office.

Today Feng Shui is used widely around the world, seeing value in what the Chinese have known for years and the objectives vary depending on the home or business owners desired outcome. The common desired outcomes include; healthy family relationships, improved **physical and mental health, preservation or growth of financial wealth and harmony. When we consider the energy we put out and take in, and apply the**

Feng Shui principles, we discover that we have more control over our lives than we originally believed. Feng Shui is our opportunity to direct the flow of energy in our lives as we choose. For those of you looking for a way to bring more success for wellness into your life, you can use the basics of Feng Shui to help you achieve your goal.

This book contains tips provided in a manner through harnessing the positive energies that you and your property can receive through the use of Feng Shui principles.

Invite your desired health in

Feng Shui is a science that works beyond the physical world of cause and effect, operating on an energetic level to bring you the highest levels of good fortune. Using Feng Shui principles you create a better flow of energy in your environment and consciously direct that flow to achieve the wellness you desire in your life.

The positive energy of an environment surrounds you and influences you 24 hours a day, seven days a week, your whole lifetime, this also applies to uncured negative energy. Feng Shui is like a form of acupuncture or bar codes for the unified field of energy that includes your home and body. Activate or cure areas within your home or workplace and you start a flow of energy through your body, mind, and soul for more success in your career, health, relationships and growth.

Brain Waves- Your home or workspace is a living, vibrating energy in a vast unified field of energy. Everything in a home influences the flow of active and passive energy also known as positive or negative Qi. This energy wave of flow is similar to the brainwaves formed from your own thinking process. The outcomes in your life are results of brain waves you habitually create with your thoughts. And the outcomes you experience in life are either suppressed or enhanced by the energy fields or environmental brainwaves emitting in your physical surroundings.

There are two brainwave energy fields or environmental brainwaves are beta and alpha frequencies. Beta frequencies reflect chaos and are present in cluttered rooms, drab, dirty spaces, environments with no cosiness or spaces filled with depressing or violent images, dead flowers and piles of papers. This environment feels overwhelming and joyless. It produces victim mentality where one feels unsupported. It creates the feeling of struggling uphill. In this state it is very hard to create what you want toward a better life. However, when you begin to declutter and clean the spaces. Introduce colours and uplifting images, the beta energy wave's shift to bring in the flow of alpha brainwaves. You invite in new opportunities and attract more of the power available to you. This positive flow brings to you good fortune in your career, relationships, health and growth as well as feeling more empowered.

Feng Shui has shown through the centuries that improving your success is within your control. When you change or add other things such as colours or items or position yourself or your furniture, this creates a positive spiralling of energy upward that affects your good fortune and you are in a much better position to attract what you desire. When you decide what you want or to make a change in your life the first thing you must do is get rid of the old to make room for the new. If you want good health for your loved ones and yourself, you must make room, change or add something to invite it in.

General Space Feng Shui is universal. Each of the eight compass directions, plus the center direction, is associated with a specific life area, element, number, shape, material, colour, and symbol. Some of the directions include a representative season and animal. Any area can be activated by placing specific elements, colours, items or images, in the specific compass direction and area of your home or workplace.

Compass directions for Health, including your loved ones, home and you are north for clarity and self-empowerment. South for balance and celebration. East for general health, central health, focus and honesty. West for purity, transparency and joy. Northwest for transformation and faith. Northeast for harmony Southwest for compassion and Southeast for forgiveness and release.

Decluttering and cleaning is the start in creating a flow of positive Qi. By placing items and images you activate environmental affirmations that represent what it is you want to have happen in this area of your life. These environmental affirmations are your physical visualisation board. Every time you look at your items or objects you are sending the Qi in this direction, consciously and unconsciously

Feng Shui for health is a priority to consider when looking to apply Feng shui principles to your home or workplace. If your or your family's health is out of balance, the negative flow of Qi in your environment plays a key factor in creating this and can appear as: for an extended period you have complications with your health and have tried different doctors, medicines, or therapies with little long-term benefit, have been hospitalised or had major surgery since you moved into a new home or office building, or illness keeps recurring. If you would like to invite wellness, attract the right solutions for maintaining your health or enhance and maintain what you already experience Feng shui can help increase your energy levels and help increase the flow of positive Qi for wellness to enter into your experience as well as creating a good foundation for continued wellness.

Clutter management

Letting go of the past is Forgiveness as is letting go of things that have negative connections or serve no worthwhile purpose. This makes space for positive replacements. Feng Shui recognises that clutter can make people feel disorganised, uncreative, tired, anxious and burdened. Energy or Qi is all around us, all the time, the clutter is a clutter of energies. And this affects our health.

Positive Qi, can become blocked by clutter. When energy is blocked, it becomes stagnate and then turns to negative energy. That is why one of the main principles of Feng Shui is that you must de-clutter your home. It's important to remember that getting rid of the old makes way for the new.

Start by clearing out everything that doesn't need to be there, unload it. In order to get new things in your life you have to release old things. Look around your home. Let go of Failure. If you have health problems, let go broken and rusty items, as well as anything that represents lack of health. Let go of anything representing your previous illnesses such as x-rays, doctor's reports or diaries with medical appointments. Put them all in a box and store it somewhere to tell the universe there is space for a renewed success. Let go of everything, even old images, particularly ones where you or your loved ones are unwell. Release it all. If you do not have much time to clean and clear presently, place in closed spaces, or boxes and cover the boxes with beautiful fabrics. When clutter is visible, your sub conscious mind sends a message of chaos to the universe.

Sometimes it can be challenging to get rid of things that we don't need, but in doing so, we free up more of our energy to devote to the things we want. If you resist letting go of items because you spent money on them, you are holding on to old energy patterns that block your Qi moving forward and your resistance is indicating lack and limitation, and you are not ready to move forward to your ideal health. Even holding onto things for a later date, or just in case is indicating lack and limitation, as well as inviting some adversity to occur.

Here's an example: When we apply the best quality make-up this will not help the skin look healthy in the long term. If the skin is not cleansed and taken care of properly by using the correct procedures and products such as cleansers and good foods it will not stay vibrant and healthy. It also invites conditions to amplify unhealthy skin. It's the same concept with clutter in your home. If you carry all that old clutter around, blocking the flow and not taking care of it, there is no room in your life for new things to prosper. Success will pass you by because you're too busy holding on to lack and clutter.

Release and remove any images, items or paperwork of poor health by replacing them with something more uplifting and vibrant. Remove anything that reminds you of previous ill health such as something you received while in hospital. Even music can have an affect particularly if it is a song that reminds you of the time you were unwell. Letting go of that which does not contribute to your health and happiness makes room for new health, happiness and fulfilment.

Your living areas

Represent the present. Too much clutter creates stagnant Qi as well as inconvenience and frustration. Remove items that are from previous ailments or items given to you that you do not particularly like. Place something that makes you feel good and makes you smile. Lilac represents the frequency of releasing, use lavender oils in your soaps, lotions and cleaning products to cleanse the stagnant, dense Qi.

Activate your Home or Office For in Health

Outside areas

Represents the present. Clear gardens of dried plants, or rubbish lying around, clean paths and maintain this, it allows the flow of positive Qi to enter. No faded, broken items or dried plants, the positive Qi is not present in these.

The Basement or under your home/office

Represents the past. This is better place to store things, however, too much stored indicates you are trapped in the past.

The attic

Represents the future. Too much stored here can block your future and the futures of generations to come. Avoid storage above the bedrooms or lounge room.

Improve your Qi flow with FORGIVENSS and RELEASE

- Let go of possessions, emotions, and thoughts that keep you stuck.
- The colour violet represents forgiveness
- Elevate the level of Qi in your environment and yourself.
- Let go of photos, objects, and furnishings from your past that no longer serve you
- Reliving old memories is stagnant Qi. Let go of the past, things that have no allocated space or serve no worthwhile purpose. Remember that getting rid of the old makes way for the new Qi.

Move on to make new, happy healthy memories. Free up the stuck, dense energy to create a brilliant future

- Have a more positive outlook and focus on the things you are grateful for. Start a gratitude journal. Each day write three things you are grateful for.

- Antiques can have mental, emotional, and even spiritual impressions attached to them, release the dense Qi of the past by using lavender, geranium, and rosemary essential oils added to water for cleaning.

- Clear and organise your home or workspace to get the energy flowing, and prepare for wellness, new experiences, and opportunities into your life. Create space for good fortune to enter your life by creating an uncluttered space in every room.

.

Activate your wellness

A Feng Shui consultant uses the combination of Space Feng Shui and Time Feng Shui.

Space Feng Shui assessments determine the directions Qi flows in and around your physical environment. This includes General space orientation and activation of the home or office as well as activating and enhancing Personal Space Feng Shui based on an individual's Personal fortune directions to improve/increase Success, Health, Relationships and Growth. Time Feng Shui is the analysis of time cycles or Visiting Energy Assessments and the nature of specific energy flows of time cycles. All have their appointed compass direction, each of these nine directions have significant purposes, and the east including the centre of your home or workplace is your general health sector.

Personal fortune directions or Personal Space Feng Shui as mentioned above can only be assessed on an individual basis where a person's birthdate and other factors are required for accurate assessment. General Space Feng Shui is universal, the following pages contain general space health to self practice.

Feng Shui and quantum physics teaches that everything in our physical environment carries an energy that is moving our lives forward in that direction. By placing in our physical surroundings objects or images that have a positive personal meaning, we are activating and sending the Qi in this direction every time we look at it. Even if we think we do not see it any longer, it is still registering the message on a sub-conscious level.

General Health
Your health is associated to the overall energy of the whole environment, however, there are two areas that are connected

on a deeper energy level for the state of your well-being. They are the centre and east direction of your home or workplace.

Based on Feng Shui principles, how healthy is your environment, how healthy is your bedroom. What is the quality of air in your home or workplace? Many homes and workplaces contain low and stagnant energy. And this affects wellness in many ways.

The East direction represents general health. The element is Wood and is symbolised by the Green Dragon. Place a proud dragon figure or image here to enhance health. Ensure you place it where you can see it and that the dragon is lower than eye level so it does not overpower you. Include live plants to enhance the wood energy. The Qi or life-force of the plant, will energise the space as well as naturally removing indoor toxins and purify the air you breathe. Dead plants and dried flowers are a source of negative energy. If the plant is not blossoming, do not leave it sitting in your room to stagnate the flow you're trying to create.

If you or your family often gets ill, place a small water fountain in the lounge or family room, water nourishes the wood element.

The Centre

The center of your home is considered very important, because it is from the center that all other areas of your environment draw their energy nourishment. The center is called the heart of the home, or the yin yang point. The more open and happy the center of the home is, the happier, more open and healthier the people who live in that home tend to be.

Also the centre of the home or workspace represents balance between all the elements, Earth, Metal, Water, Wood and Fire. It relates to health issues, spirituality and whether you feel energised with a sense of life balance and wellbeing. If you feel unwell, overwhelmed, stressed and lacking in vitality this is the area to concentrate on. Keep it clutter free and place a clear crystal quartz here for harmony.

Create a wonderful balance for your health by adding an activation to the center of each space in your home or workplace. Place rocks, crystals, ceramics, candles, metal objects, plants and clear, clean glass objects. Do not activate in the bathroom. These are drain areas, this tells the Universe you are flushing it all away. Always close the bathroom door and ensure the toilet lid is down to keep the flushing energy from connecting with the higher level energy in the rest of your spaces. Take good care of your center by creating vibrant and harmonious energy there, place happy items and images, what happiness means to you and your loved ones.

Never place tall column objects such as tall bookshelves or tall lamps in the center of your home or office. These items represent a tree that is digging into the earth or a metal rod digging out the earth, much like a shovel, both uprooting and disturbing the earth, this indicates disruption to your health.

When buying or remodelling a home, avoid spiral staircases, this drains energy very quickly. A spiral staircase represents a whirlwind funnel that sucks up everything and uproots everything in its path. If you have this in your home or workplace, enclose it with a wall or screens.

Quality of air

We are fed by the air we breathe and the impact of our surroundings. The environment is influenced by the level of Qi in a room, breathing clean air regularly is a foundation for your health and well-being. Fresh, good quality air is often ignored, and this is a Feng shui health priority. Aerate your spaces to bring in new fresh Qi and replace recycled air. Ensure you maintain high levels of Qi by opening windows and doors wide and often, do whatever it takes to find solutions for better air in your home. An oil burner, incense, ioniser or air purifier will enhance the positive flow. Ensure the air you breathe is clean.

Natural light

This also includes indoor lighting. Once you focus on the quality of light in your environment you will feel a positive shift in your health and well-being. Light as well as colour are our nutrients, particularly sunlight. Give your environment and body enough light nutrition. If any spaces are limited with natural light ensure that you use lamps in the dark areas. All the four corners of each room in your home or workspace should be well-lit. Dark areas and corners create dense, negative Qi. If you are unable to light all four corners of each space, ensure that every corner of your living room has light. If you have fluorescent light bulbs, replace them if possible, they increase electromagnetic energy that interferes with health use LED lights or lamps instead of the general lighting if these are fittings in your home. Also place in your home or workspace vibrant art, ensure it is happy and joyful with fresh, alive colours. Be it a wall colour, art or fresh flowers, your energy is strengthened by the presence of colour and light.

Clear space

As stated in the previous chapter clutter clearing is essential for creating a positive flow of Qi. All activations including colours, objects or plants will negate against the low, depressing energy of clutter. Unclutter your spaces, cupboards and drawers, available space invites free flowing Qi. Clutter constantly drains energy from you. Open, clean, clear and organised space welcomes new opportunities and invites room for your health to improve, flourish and thrive.

Set your Intention

Clearly visualise your life with your ideal health goal. Write this in a journal. Write in the now as though you are watching a movie about it. The stronger and clearer you are in stating what you'd like, the easier it is for the universe to send you your heart's desire. Write a list of all the qualities perfect health is to you and in the positive. Is it vitality, clear skin, a certain weight, great posture, walking with ease? What do you feel like? How would that look, feel, taste, smell? Bring that sense into your home with specific images, colours, and scents that reflect the energy you want. Do not place sad or dark images. Place images and items that represent vibrancy and good health to send the message of wellness such as clear, clean glass to represent clear, clean health.

Areas in the environment

To have relationships that are loving and supportive at all times is a blessing. To have a healthy, beautiful and happy environment to share with your loved ones is to be blessed twice.

The art and science of Feng Shui is intricate and complex. Houses and their surroundings are studied carefully for their influence on people living in the house. Our environments are powerful energy attractors that may or may not be serving what it is we truly want to bring into our experience The quality of energy in your environment determines the quality of your health and when Feng Shui principles are implemented, this creates positive energy flow in the environment bringing more peace and vitality for all members, both young and old.

When improvements are made to the east and centre health direction of your surroundings in combination with improvements made to the complementing areas, you could live a long and healthy life. Health is the center of the Bagua (eight trigrams, or eight compass directions) and touches all other areas of the Bagua, just as your health touches all aspects of your life. Good health must be priority. Only in good health are you able to enjoy your relationships with friends and loved ones, travel , be creative, have children, or enjoy your wealth..

By incorporating Feng Shui principles you can create a peaceful, harmonious space, allowing the energy to flow in a positive manner. When your home is a relaxed one, your mood will reflect this, and you in turn will become more relaxed and less stressed. Stress is responsible for so many ailments. As the stress disappears, the ailments will too. Practice Feng shui in your workplace to create a space that encourages relaxation as well as productivity.

Lounge/Family Room

The energy of family health and harmony is closely connected to the family bagua area of your home. Place in the east direction elements of vibrant wood, a fountain for positive Qi flow, as well as happy family photos.

The primary element of the Health direction is earth. Place a potted plant in a ceramic pot to improve or maintain good health, yellow daisies in a white ceramic vase can help brighten up your room as well as your spirits. Enhance with some fire elements here because fire helps to create earth. Place little candles in the center of your coffee table or dining table.

Dining Room

Hang a mirror with a gold frame reflecting the dining table. Keep fresh fruit or flowers on the table. This brings life, energy, and invites good health and is doubled by the mirror.

Bedroom

Most people spend one third of their lives in a bedroom, some such as teenagers can spend more. This area requires focus on creating good energy flow for your well-being, as well as the quality of your intimate relationship.

The bedroom is for rest, rejuvenation and romance. Ensure your bed and bedroom support this. Position the bed where the headboard is against a solid wall and that you can clearly see the entry door. Avoid placing the bed in line with a doorway, since this can cause feelings of vulnerability and defensiveness. Also avoid alignment with the bathroom door, as this can contribute to feeling drained, tired or having restless sleep patterns.

Do not sleep under a window. Moonlight on the head, brings lack of focus during the daytime. Ensure your bed has balanced energy on both sides for example do not have one side of the bed up against a wall. Ensure both sides of the bed have a side table, light and a pleasant view. Position other furniture harmoniously. Good furniture arrangements play a significant role in Feng Shui. It is important to have a clear path to enter your bedroom, no matter what section of the house it's located in. Try to make sure that large furniture is not placed too near the doorway.

Avoid storing a lot of electronics in bedrooms. The constant hum of electricity and blinking lights disrupts the flow of energy, and it is difficult to relax in that environment even when you are asleep. If you must have electronics in the room, be sure to put them away when you're not using them. Place alarm clocks at least 5 or 6 feet away from body unless they run on batteries.

Ensure you do not have a mirror reflecting the bed. A mirror that reflects your image when you are in bed scatters thoughts and create negative dreams, it also doubles any health problems you may have. It's best to avoid putting a television in the room, this affects the energy in the room, and it also reflects the bed. If you choose to have this, place a cover over it when not in use.

Ensure items in the room have a proper place. There must also be order to the room. Visual symmetry provides peace of mind, and it keeps the energy flowing through the room evenly.

Do not put water in the room, actual water or images with water, this attracts more unsettling dreams. No live plants or flowers because they have too much active yang energy for the bedroom, calm yin energy is required.

Avoid work related items or exercise equipment. The bedroom is a passive space, not yang energy. Place your work desk or computer elsewhere. If you have no other place to for a home office ensure the computer and all the work related items are put away before going to bed so you do not see it from your bed The also applies to exercise equipment, place it elsewhere, not under the bed otherwise the active energy will promote a restless sleep.

Exposed beams over a bed and a part of the body, creates problems in that area. When sleeping under a beam people have problems because these structures put pressure on their aura. Beams straight across over the head symbolises the guillotine and good energy will be cut off before it benefits you. Thin and sharp beams have greater impact than beams that are flat and wide. Diagonal beams indicate that the good energy will start to flow but will not finish right. Sitting under beams for several hours has the same effect as sleeping under beams. Move your bed if it is under a beam. If your space is limited and your bed cannot be moved, cover the beam with fabric or paint the beam to match the ceiling. No see through fabric.

Sleeping in a room where the street traffic faces you directly is a negative Feng Shui situation. The lights of the cars represent the eyes of the tiger stalking and attacking you, this creates stress. Place window coverings such as heavy curtains to block out the lights and hang a pakua mirror on the outside of the window. These are special 8-sided mirrors used to cure negative Qi.

Allow natural light in during the day, and good air flow. Do not store anything under the bed, and keep your wardrobes clean and organised.

Ensure you have a solid headboard this represents support, and energetically brings both sides of the bed together, creating harmonious union. If possible, avoid metal bedframes they enhance the water element and water should never be in the bedroom, metal is yang Qi and attracts unsettling dreams.

Too much stuff piled in a bedroom (or any room for that matter) is a huge energetic distraction that subconsciously pulls us away from our focus. The bedroom is a space for rest, rejuvenation and relief from the outside world. Remove the clutter such as computers, exercise equipment, paperwork, kids' projects, or piled clothes, find a place for them. Just be careful not to clutter up another part of your home, everything must have its place or it is considered as clutter.

Hang a six tube metal wind chime or a crystal in the center of the bedroom to enhance the energy in the space.

Make your bed, every morning it shapes the day for success transforming chaos into order. And since we spend a third of our lives in bed, this enhances devotion to yourself.

Feng Shui principles in children's rooms creates a healthy, loving and safe environment. A child's room created with Feng Shui applications will serve as an emotional and physical support during the experiences of your child's growth as well as harmonise their relationships. How healthy and fresh is the air your child breathes in? How much natural light does your child get? What is the quality of artificial lights in your child's room?

Considering the presence of all electrical appliances, what is the level of electromagnetic energy your child is exposed to? What is the level of clutter in the room? A good energy foundation in your children's rooms is very important. Ensure your child's bedroom is a clean, clutter free space for positive energy to flow easily. Also allow fresh air to enter and position the bedhead to a solid wall.

Your bedroom, bathroom and kitchen are your home trinity, ensure they are clean and uncluttered with no expired products. This will reflect in the energy of your health if it one or more are left unattended.

Bathroom and Kitchen

Remove any expired products from the fridge, pantry and bathroom cabinets, including expired health supplements and medications. Place fresh fruit on display, and place health supplements in the east area of your kitchen.

Clutter management in the bathroom and kitchen is required as in all other areas in your environment. Ensure your kitchen stove and refrigerator are clean, orderly, and also in good working order. Do not let dirty dishes pile up.

Activate your Home or Office For in Health

Fire placement in our environment affects our physical self and our homes health and longevity. If a stove or fireplace is incorrectly placed then it can bring sickness, financial problems and misfortune. When fire is correctly placed it can support the health, prosperity and status of your. Kitchens are vital to a home's overall health. The placement of your appliances is more important than the actual direction your kitchen faces, because incorrect appliance placement can create negative Qi. A fire placement analysis of your kitchen is advisable. This assessment includes Personal fortune directions or Personal Space Feng Shui and can only be assessed on an individual basis where a person's birthdate and other factors are required for accurate assessment. General Space Feng Shui is universal, if you have an oven in the east or north direction of your kitchen place a bowl of still water to reduce the effects of ill health. If the stove and sink are directly opposite or in line with each other, hang a Pakua crystal between them. However, it is recommended that you appoint a Feng Shui Consultant for exact analysis. Place potted plants or herbs in the East direction of the kitchen to enhance Qi flow.

Drains in sinks of the bathroom or kitchen can wash away positive Qi. Plugging sinks with rubber stoppers when they are not in use to prevents the new flow of energy from flowing down the drain. You can also use rocks or pebbles instead of a rubber stopper. The rocks help form a barricade and create a pleasing aesthetic. Also keep the toilet lid down and the bathroom door closed.

Keep brooms and mops stored in closets and pantry doors closed at all times. These items are used to clean up dense negative Qi.

It's very important that the doors in the kitchen do not lead directly into the front or back doors. This kind of alignment means the Qi energy rushes through the kitchen and out of the house. When this kind of placement occurs, it creates unbalanced Qi that brings illnesses and misfortunes to those in the home. Place a mirror at the entrance of the kitchen.

Ensure that your bathroom is clean, and organised and has a sense of beauty and pampering energy. Do not place photographs of friends or family members, as well as awards. These are drain areas, this tells the Universe you are flushing it all away. Your well-being is intricately connected to the quality of energy in your bathroom. Create a spa feel that pleases your senses, add a pleasant smell, soft soap, soft bath linens, candles, an aromatherapy diffuser, or any other items that can help create a spa feeling in your bathroom.

Front Door

Your entry point is also known as the mouth of Qi, and this includes your front door. It is the energy connection of your home. It is where the Qi enters along with what you and others bring or take with you. When you leave, you take what you're feeling with you into your day. When you come home, you bring in all that has happened to you throughout the day. The first priority for your mouth of Qi is to clear the clutter from around your door. If you and your family store shoes, coats, equipment, toys, or any other items by the front door, move them. The clutter blocks the free flow of energy, and prevents it from entering your life.

In Feng shui, the view you first see as you open your front door is very important, as is the view from your bed. They set the energy your body is receiving throughout the day. Ensure your eyes have views that make you feel good.

Workspace

Wind chimes attract good chi. Hang a wind chime over your desk or work space to increase positive Qi flow. Ensure that it is a six-rod hollow metal wind chime. This wind chime is the best moving metal activator because it removes the density of the negative Qi in its hollow tubes and six is the energetic number for metal. There are no substitutions for using these wind chimes. For example, bells do not work. You can also hang wind chimes in windows that you open frequently to invite abundance into your home or workspace.

Outside Areas

Outside areas follow the same principals as the inside environment. The health sector is located in the center and east corner of the yard. Ensure that the yard is properly trimmed and cleared of rubbish. Plant a garden and install a fountain or a fish pond. You can also include other symbols of health, such as a wind chime. Place white flowers in the area, this creates purity in health. You can use many of the same activations you used for the health sectors inside your home.

Body/Home Connection

Every part of the home is connected with a part of the body. Impurity in any of these areas create problems to the related body part.

Face

The entrance to the home. Keep it clean for better working senses, lack of Qi in your entrance brings facial pains or skin problems. Never place wastebaskets at the entrance, because Qi stagnates around clutter.

Hands and feet

Represent the four corners of the home:

Hands - the two front corners

Feet - the two back corners.

A messy storage place in any corner relates to these body parts. Hands and feet also represent how you walk into life and handle yourself in the world– the cleaner the four corners of the home, the stronger your position in the world.

Heart

The Centre of the home also known as the heart, it can also be any favourite room. Keep this area clean and tidy and without obstruction.

Kidney

The Bathroom represents the kidneys. If you have kidney problems, check your bathroom for clues.

Liver

The Kitchen represents the liver. Remove old food and expired products from your cabinets and fridge. Use fresh dish cloths and good smelling products to clean the kitchen. A cluttered kitchen means the liver works overtime and does not eliminate the toxins.

Pancreas and Abundance

The Dining room table represents the pancreas as well as abundance. Keep it clean and ready for the next meal. Do not use it for storage or clutter

Lungs

Glass in doors and windows represent the lungs. Keep windows clean to breathe easier.

Intestines

The Hallways represent the intestines. Keep hallways clear to encourage the flow of positive Qi.

Spine and bones

The structure of the home represents the spine and bones. When your porch leans, roof sags, or foundation heaves, it is felt in the bones.

Learning to nurture yourself and balance giving with receiving are imperative. Nourish and strengthen your energy. Crystals and gemstones help support your energy and enhance vitality. Wearing these as jewellery or having crystals in your home are good ways to benefit from their energy.

Working with essential oils can also help balance and nourish your energy. Choose from a variety of oils that calm, strengthen and balance, such as chamomile or lavender, or the ones that energise and revitalize, such as lemongrass or eucalyptus. Use them in your bedroom, in your lounge room, and even in your car.

Look after yourself through maintaining a healthy, balanced eating habit and exercise. Exercise does not need to be rigorous, try Qigong, Tai Chi or yoga. Add supplements to your daily oral intake, this adds the nutrients we require that are not received from produce and preservatives in many consumables in the marketplace these days. Please note: Not all supplements are pure, ensure you look for the ones that are derived from the natural source with no chemical additives. Also listen to some guided meditations. If you are stressed and your energy is imbalanced, take a deep breath through your nose, hold it for a couple of seconds and release it out from your mouth, go for a walk in the fresh air or change what you are doing, this is a great way to hit the reset button in your situation in the moment. A reset will help you to think logically about your situation and formulate a plan to lessen the emotional impact, this enables you to work towards a resolution or to establish whether it deserves your escalated emotional level. Avoid being consumed by negative emotions such as anger or despair, your health will be negatively impacted as a result. Do something that will make you feel good.

Geopathic stress

"Geo" means "Earth" or "Land", "Pathic" indicates both a disease, as well as a cure for disease. It also indicates the ability to feel, perceive or be sensitive to specific energies as in telepathic. There are various types of earth energies, some are very good for health, and some are detrimental. These include: Earth magnetic grid lines, underground flowing water, sewer and grey water pipes, electromagnetic frequency (EMF), radio frequency and microwaves. Geopathic stress acts on the body's energy field to weaken the immune system. This can reduce the state of our health. There are indications that someone may be suffering the effects of geopathic stress, these include: Poor sleeping patterns, particularly waking in the morning to feel that you have not had a proper night's sleep, grinding of teeth during the night, unexplained headaches, displays of severe impatience and anger, a grey 'unwashed' pallor and, often, very lifeless hair, and low energy levels

Place an Ionizer: Ionic Air Purifier, salt lamp or amethyst crystal in your spaces. These are great at generating negative ions from moisture in the air. This crystal can be worn too. Clean areas with lavender products and enhance with lavender essential oil in Harmonisers/burners.

Avoid metal bed frames and spring mattresses, they bundle and reflect geopathic energies. They also charge easily from electro-magnetic fields. Replace with wooden frames and latex or foam mattress.

We are surrounded by electromagnetic activity that can magnify geopathic stress. High tension power lines, satellite towers, electric poles, or circuit breakers all send out high and low frequency energy that can increase geopathic stress, as can everyday items like microwaves, cell phones, and wireless routers. Minimise your exposure to such devices, get rid of unneeded appliances. Unplug them when not in use.

Ensure that bedrooms are as free as possible from electromagnetic activity. Remove some or all electrical devices such as television, phones, computers, electric alarm clocks, and kindles.

Cleansing
Energy can neither be created nor destroyed; rather, it

transforms from one form to another. When unpleasant feelings linger, space cleansing the environment transforms the energy to positive Qi leaving it lighter, healthier and happier, this creates more success. Everything that happens in an environment including conflict, trauma, and illness leave imprints and can attract other unwanted dense energy unless they are intentionally cleared. Subtle traces of past events can make places feel happy or sad. Replacing old carpet or furnishings, clutter management and redecorating all help to transform the negative dense Qi as well as cleaning the environment with lavender oils. Place a few drops of lavender oil in your cleaning products.

Express Happiness

Quantum physics states like attracts like energy. A home that is clean, clutter free and loved will attract and promote harmony and happiness. Organise your home so that everything has its place. Most importantly, express love and care with all your home contents, this indicates good support, care, happiness and well-being of your family. Create a home that is beautiful, joyful and full of love

General

Walk around your home or workspace. Are you stopped by furniture or do you stumble on a rug? Do you have a hard time opening doors? Air should flow around everything in your home. Move furniture away from walls, even if just a couple of inches. Pull furniture pieces together to create an area where air can flow around. Use your windows. Windows should never be blocked. Natural light is very important and brings with it positive energy.

In the practice of Feng Shui, mirrors are used to reflect energy into other areas of the home, ensure mirrors are not reflecting doors, it will bounce the energy back out. Mirrors require proper placement, they can dramatically shift the flow of energy in any given space. Mirrors also bring a sense of refreshment and calm. Direct the flow of Qi with mirrors, lights, plants, colours, and items. Some obstacles are good, because they slow rushing Qi and enhance Feng Shui, however, some are bad, because they collect and spread stagnant Qi. Sense whether the obstacles feel good or bad. To direct the flow of energy down a hall to rooms such as the sleeping areas or workspace, hang a mirror or an image with reflective glass opposite the door to each room. When an obstacle blocks the flow of Qi, such as a plant, place a mirror so that it can reflect the energy toward thee direction you want the Qi to flow.

There can be many subtle factors in an environment that supports us with either positive or negative results in our health. Awareness and observation can move you from the negative to the positive flow.

Add indoor plants and trees whenever you want growth or better health. Avoid the cactus, as spikes invite criticism when grown inside. The Qi or life-force of the plant, will energise the space as well as naturally remove indoor toxins and purify the air we breathe. Just remember that dead plants are a source of negative energy. If you would like to cook healthier meals more often place a plant in your kitchen or if you want to be more productive at work, plants on your desk or home office bring positive, creative energy to your work environment.

Add some motion to a space that is stuck. A stuck space usually reflects a stuck life. Move things around the room this helps liven the atmosphere. The Feng shui number to help guide you through this process of getting unstuck is twenty-seven. Just by moving twenty-seven things around a space whether it's a paper clip or a desk can bring positive energy to a room that was previously lacking it.

The west is the area of purity and communication. Enhance this direction in your lounge/family room with items or pictures related to children such as children playing, or family pictures of you with your children. You can also place an item or image of a laughing Buddha to increase happiness. If you work with children, also activate the West direction in your workplace with pictures of the children you work with or care for.

Along with structure, items and colours your words create your environment. Something as subtle and innocent as a word enters our subconscious and affects how we feel. Be conscious on your vocabulary, and watch it shape your path. When we honour ourselves with good words, including praise for ourselves and others, we fuel our ability to live a good life.

Your Personal Fortune Directions and Time Feng Shui for Money and Success

Your Personal Fortune directions are based on your Kua number, and has a greater effect for you personally than general space Feng Shui. The areas include success, relationships, health and growth, and is established by gender, as well as date of birth. When you know your Personal Fortune Directions you can face it for added success in health, as well as place activations in these directions to amplify your personal successes. There are four misfortune directions as well. When you are aware of these directions you can cure and ensure specific placements are not hindering your success. To establish the fortune colour, element, shape and fabric for your wellness and other aspects requires a Personal Fortune direction analysis, a Feng Shui Consultant is recommended.

Never place anything into your space that you do not love just because you are told you to do so. Feng Shui is about creating a positive flow of Qi as well as creating a living space that feeds your soul and uplifts your spirits. Objects you don't love will have the opposite effect. The more personal the objects are to you, the more Qi they will generate. Representations of items do not require to be only one thing such as Eastern symbols. An example is the Chinese symbolism for a tortoise, the Celestial Guardian of the North, this can be represented by any tortoise, live, image or object.

Health enhancers

Feng Shui cures obstacles, strengthens intentions and addresses how the Qi flows through an environment. A value of Feng Shui is to bring our awareness to those areas of our life which are not in harmony with our intention. There are several approaches to making these adjustments and enhancements by adjusting the home or workplace environment, even ourselves. We can remove negative Qi and other dense factors that distract, slow down or, in some other way, divert our intention for desired health.

The Bagua directions of a home or workplace divides the structure or individual spaces into nine areas of life activity and these are connected by distinct energy fields of the spaces along with objects, images, plants animals and people. Through people and animals emotions and personal practises are also emitted. When you improve the energy of your home, you change yourself and your life and by applying the Feng Shui principles for self enhancement you evolve to fulfil your desires. Author *Napoleon Hill* explains, *"Our brains become magnetised with the dominating thoughts which we hold in our minds, and, by means with which no man is familiar, these 'magnets' attract to us the forces, the people, the circumstances of life which harmonise with the nature of our dominating thoughts."*

CLARITY

Clarity is the quality of being easily understood, expressed, remembered and of being easily seen or heard

Feng Shui principles assist you in communicating more clearly in your health intentions by expressing your needs and desires openly, earnestly and wholly. Through establishing and applying your desires in your environment it creates impressive results from your efforts and avoids misunderstandings.

Clarity begins with deciding what you want. What kind of wellness. How do you see good health? Prioritise areas where you require fast results. Determine exactly what you want to accomplish. Bring a clear, accurate message of your desired outcome for your health and wellness. Place symbols, images or objects reflecting the outcome that you want to create. Let go of images that no longer clearly represent your intentions. Take care of what has not been completed now, just by starting and ticking off even your simplest tasks invites the positive Qi of clarity.

To send the best message about abundance in wellness and invite clarity, clean water features. Light up your home, workplace, yard and entry. Add bright objects and plants. Place happy items an images in the eight directions including the Centre of your home or workspace that represent vitality, freshness and joy.

Ensure the entrance to your home or workplace has clear messages showing the world to recognise and respond to your personality or business also indicating that a very successful person is inside. Also Place happy items or images outside. Do not hang dark or depressing images.

CELEBRATION

South stands for fame and recognition as well as music, celebration, and festivity, activate the South area by placing orange objects in lounge room or workplace. Unless you want to get pregnant do not activate celebration in the bedroom.

Celebrate your efforts and accomplishments, changes, significant dates and celebrate yourself! Cooked a great meal, celebrate, completed your tasks, celebrate. Add the positive flow of celebration to anything you choose to rejoice for.

Manifest more joy showing off your awards and place them in gold frames to invite abundance. This will give you more to celebrate.

Celebrate your accomplishments by throwing a party. Do not wait for others. Create celebrations for yourself. Feng Shui is a consistent celebration of positive flowing Qi. Include children in your parties, because they represent the fortune of the family.

If you want to have a baby make space for your baby by clearing the clutter under the bed. Elephants are considered a wish-granting animal. Place a pair of wooden elephants on both sides of your bedroom door as if they were walking into the room, so they make your wish walk through that same door. Also place an image of children or a stuffed animal in the west direction of your bedroom to invite energies supportive of conception and birth.

To heal a broken heart use orange essential oils. This is considered as a natural antidepressant and an effective treatment for emotional downs. The oil is used to bring peace and calm to an emotional situation while inviting serenity and harmony. Add orange essential oil to a spray bottle filled with water, and spray around your spaces each day. Ancient wisdom praises the use of oranges to help peel away your problems. Place the peels from the oranges, plus two cups of Epsom salts, into a bath and soak in it. Your enthusiasm and optimism will return.

The TRINITY of LUCK

In Feng Shui, there are three categories which describe the type of luck we experience in our lives, they are:

Heaven Luck- This refers to the karma, destiny, health types, astrological horoscope and the family environment you were born into and is determined by the cycles of time. This type of luck cannot be controlled. You can however, through astrological cycles or the Chinese Astrology Almanac, also known as the Tung Shu prepare for times when you are more likely to experience positive and negative points towards key areas in your life such as health, relationships, career, or finances. It helps to take note of astrological periods. This indicates where your key life lessons will be more likely to occur. Your astrological chart also helps determine areas where you are more likely to experience luck potential. These astrological events can affect communications, contractual problems, delays, travel, machinery breakdown and times of change and unexpected news. To make the most of your overall luck potential, you should develop a positive, progressive attitude while applying Feng Shui principles to your home and work environment, as well as keeping up to date with major astrological changes in your life. Luck is ultimately when skill and knowledge, plus the right attitude, meet opportunity. Feng Shui can help the flow of Qi that attracts positive energy, this increases your abundance opportunities.

Earth Luck - This type of luck is determined by our surroundings for example our home or workspace and the way in which we direct ourselves with positive or negative energy combinations, within and around the earth. This type of luck can be improved and enhanced when Feng Shui is correctly applied to your home or work environment. It deals with balance, element cycles, mathematical probability factors, magnetic orientation, surrounding landform and time dimensional analysis.

Human Luck - This refers to your personal attitude, education, managerial and financial ability, lifestyle, virtues, the choices that you make and your personal quest for knowledge. As an individual, you have full control over this type of luck, and when it is combined with Earth Luck through the correct application of Feng Shui, you increase your experience for greater harmony, contentment and success. To truly experience the joys which life can offer, you must first examine your attitude and sense of self. Change your attitude and you can quite literally change your life. You can utilise positive symbols, words and images within your surroundings to help focus and connect your personal aspirations with the appropriate Earth Luck location combinations.

- Learn to recognise your negative self talk. We all do it to some extent. Change it to an uplifting phrase.

- The positive and negative behaviours in your life have had many years to shape you into the unique individual that you have now become. Learn to look at yourself objectively in order to recognise certain conditioned responses and patterned behaviour, this can be enlightening.

- Acknowledge each positive step that you take forward.

- Surround yourself with positive friends and family who will encourage and support you.

- Actively seek to learn and experience as much as you can from the people and environment around you. Learn from someone who has what you want. Knowledge is life with wings. Find yourself a mentor someone who you aspire to be like and admire for what they have achieved in their life. Observe the ways in which they conduct themselves.

- If you find yourself feeling negative resolve it through forgiveness. You may not alter a situation immediately, but you can take full control of your response to the situation and how you ultimately deal with it.

HONESTY and HONOUR

Honour is connected to the east and power of the dragon, a symbol of power, truth, and magic. Place Dragon Symbol or object in your workspace or lounge room lower than eye level so it does not overpower you and enjoy the Dragon's precious cosmic breath.

Improve Human Luck: Feng Shui helps create an environment to change old habits, create more self-discipline and double your talents to their full potential. HONOUR is important, Eastern cultures practice Honour.

When the flow of life is good, ride the wave. When the flow of life is not great, check to see if it is keeping you from doing what you want to do. Contemplate your behaviour. Are your actions, thoughts and feelings honourable? If not what mental programs can you change and emotions can you release.

Keep structure and good life management, practice self-help/development. These are a strong indicators of how we can change our programs. Discipline yourself to fulfil your destiny and to fully express who you are. Make it easier to stick to your intentions and actions with your family and clients. Surround yourself with people who are truthful. Be more honest with yourself and others.

Improve Heavenly Luck: Practise spiritual lessons, Qigong, yoga, prayer, meditation and positive affirmations.

Improve Earth Luck: Your environment, home and workplace, is a greater body surrounding your physical body. Every object in your home or workplace is like a cell in the greater body. And as part of the unified field of the whole, will affect your body and physical experience. There are unseen links of energy between every material thing. All part of the Quantum Physics field. This can be improved with Feng Shui practices by allowing the positive flow of Qi.

For your workspace display a pair of Fu Dogs at the entrance door to protect you against office politics and corporate power struggles.

PURITY
There are 5 levels of purity: Physical Home, office and body, Etheric, Emotional, Mental and Spiritual

Creating purity is essential if your thoughts and feelings are cluttered or chaotic, you are addicted to something or you feel abused or that people violate your boundaries.

Meditations, or exercises such as Qigong and yoga assist in creating stillness within the active mind. Visualise the light of the sun in your body and home with a light meditation. Open the windows and doors to bring in light and activate your senses. When natural light is low, use lamps in the dark areas. Ensure the four corners of each room in your home or workspace are well-lit. If you are unable to light all four corners of each space, ensure that every corner of your lounge room has light.

Clean your home or workspace with lavender oils mixed in with your cleaning products. Wash your physical body every day. Use lavender soaps or add lavender oil to your shower gel, lavender helps release toxins and old energies from your aura. Breathe air charged with negative ions, consider using an ioniser air purification system.

To invite purity into your body and new possibilities into your life, create space for what you want. Even the best activations are impeded upon in a cluttered or dirty environment, ensure you dust your furniture too.

Do not display broken objects. The life force or Qi in these objects are broken and gluing does not restore the Qi.

JOY

The West is the direction for Joy it also represents communication, and children's luck.

If you would like to appreciate everything your senses experience or you lack joy, feel sad or are depressed. Place fun, humorous items here. Add fabrics, colourful artwork, bright pillows or objects bright colours to lead eyes from colour to colour. Peach and orange are the best for joy, red and warm yellows add joy too. Activate in the lounge room for everyone to invite more joyful communication. Place joyful images, toys and smiling people. Allow more sunlight to enter the spaces and open windows to let the wind bring new Qi into the home. If you cannot open your windows, use air fresheners and burn candles. White and black colours do not create joy. Exposed beams in your entrance or lounge room can create sadness for everyone in the family, cover them in fabric or paint them the same colour as the ceiling.

TRANSPARENCY

Invite clearness of mind, body, emotions and environment. Become more organised and get your business or personal records in order

Physical transparency:

In any room or area, donate, sell, or remove everything you do not need or do not love.

Entryway: When you come home, make sure your first view is clean and uplifting. The entrance to the home is the start of the flow of Qi, so always clean the entryway even if you cannot clean the rest of the home. Do not place coats and shoes within view in the entrance. Put them away in closets or in a shoe box. Keep your rubbish bins out of sight from the entrance.

Bedroom: Make beds every morning. Hang clothes in closets.

Lounge Room and workspace: Ensure these spaces are clean and uncluttered. Clean the windows and the window coverings regularly. Vacuum pet hair from furniture and carpeting. Do not leave books, magazines, or remote controls lying around. Before going to bed, tidy up to create a fresh start for the next day.

Kitchen: Discard old food, expired products, old spices or baking ingredients. Carefully wash all kitchen surfaces. Use cleaning products with lavender essential oil. Reorganise everything that is left, from food in the fridge to the items in cupboards and drawers and on countertops.

Laundry: Ensure the room is always closed off and dirty laundry is in laundry baskets.

Dining Room: Always clean up immediately after meals and place fresh flowers or a bowl of fruit on the dining table.

Landscape: Place flowers close to the entrance. No old cars, bikes, or general rubbish lying around. Keep ornaments and garden features fresh and clean. Paint or stain the fence. Keep garden furniture and umbrella fresh and not faded. Remove sick or dead plants and trees. The positive Qi has gone from these.

General: Ensure that people can easily find the entrance and turn the light on when it is dark. Every year, place a new door mat. This mat should be solid, no holes and should not have company logos or anything that can represent you, such as your family name. This indicates others overpowering you.

Etheric transparency

The etheric field is the energy body known as the first layer in the human energy field or commonly known as the aura. This field has less dense Qi than the Qi that surrounds the physical body. This energetic body or aura is fed by the air we breathe and the impact of our surroundings. Our etheric field is influenced by the level of Qi in a room. Low energy levels of Qi create negative thoughts and depressed feelings where high energy levels of Qi help us feel raised and happy. Ensure you maintain high levels of Qi by opening windows and doors. An oil burner, incense, ioniser or air purifier will enhance the positive flow. Ensure the air you breathe is clean. Be mindful of the images, objects, and paintings you display, this can create a negative impression on you.

Emotional transparency

Emotional fields from you and your family or past inhabitants may linger in your home or workplace. There may have been a break up or constant fighting. Place a little salt and rice in all of the corners of your spaces as a gesture of abundance and gratitude and remove it after one day. Also place water with sea salt in the centre of the home or workspace for seven days.

If you are experiencing arguments this may be associated with your kitchen. If your stove is opposite a sink this indicates disharmony, fire fights with water, water boils. Hang a pakua crystal between the stove and sink to unify fire and water. Door handles can also be associated with arguments if they hit against each other. Tie a red ribbon to the handles to symbolically establish unity between these arguing door handles then cut the ribbon evenly and tie them onto the handles.

Mental transparency:

Occasional sanctuary is required in our lives, particularly when you want to put ideas into action, slow down, restore clarity or when you want to be more relaxed mentally. For mental transparency create a room with less furniture, fewer books, fewer ornaments, and fewer things to tend. It can also be a chair and window focused on a view that is spacious or a bathtub filled with essential oils and natural suds. These are vital spaces to recharge our own energetic batteries, after all we are beings that contain electricity.

Also clean your desk when you finish working to be ready for fresh ideas. Keep alarm clocks at least five feet from your head when sleeping the electrical field disturbs your sleep and interfere with your focus.

FAITH

Have strong belief and trust in yourself as well as with the ancient art of Feng Shui. Create the new energy you need to manifest your intentions. Change the way you think, feel, and act. Apply the principles and invite your chosen positive destiny to unfold. Have patience with yourself and others. Recognise the results from your Feng Shui practices. Positive and negative responses can occur as you begin making changes. Respond in a positive way, and feel relief that there is finally a logical explanation for misfortunes in your life. Feng Shui changes can stir up energy and temporarily upset order, but it will calm down as the energy finds a new order. If you resist you lose focus and concentration. Resistance leads to fear and anger, have faith in your choices.

TRANSFORMATION

Have you ever thought, if only! Or if I could turn back time. **Forgive and release the past,** say goodbye to old behaviours and beliefs that no longer serve you, and say hello to a more positive incarnation of yourself, there always has and always will be time, life offers to many wonderful opportunities, you just have to invite them in and **lay the groundwork for a better tomorrow** to welcome your new success for what you truly desire.

Boost your triumphs, live a more conscious lifestyle, get the support you need to pursue your dreams. Change the way you feel in your surroundings, change your thought patterns or how you feel about yourself and recognise your transformations.

By applying these Feng Shui practices you have placed yourself in a transformation whirlwind, a waterfall of change. Some people feel overwhelmed and disoriented, which indicates that something is changing. Things must change to allow for the new to come. *Einstein's definition of insanity, "Insanity is doing the same thing over and over again and expecting different results.".* You are sane! Stay with it and look for the positive changes from your new energy flow!

Activate your Home or Office For in Health

Ask yourself, do I feel:
Happy and more confident that everything will be all right. Peaceful in my own home. Excited about my life and the changes I want to create. Comfortable in my space and no longer running away from it. A need to change many things in my life. A sense of accomplishment because I have made more changes in one week than I have in years. Able to handle things and climb out of a depression. Open to others and myself.
How has my thinking changed? Do I feel less fear, doubt, limitation, or loneliness? Do I express more power, self-esteem, and success?

Notice the changes in your health. Perhaps you are eating healthy foods, losing weight, or playing sports. Or, you have an alternative health practitioners, started a therapy for physical improvement, meditate daily or practice Qigong.

Notice other changes such as your activity level. You might complete little jobs around the house, spend more time playing with your children or associating with friends, take up painting or writing, or express your feelings better.People around you may be offering more encouragement to pursue your dreams, or help you find the right resources.

Start a positive flow journal. Observe and record positive changes in your life. Write gratitude statements. Write in your journal daily, use blue ink, this is the colour for power. Recording your positive flow will enhance a chain of positive change in your own experiences and empower others to become active in their own good fortune and luck.

TENDERNESS

Transform your environment into a place of nurturing healing beauty, a place that has balanced energy for you and your loved ones. Be sure you genuinely love the way your spaces look and feel from wall colours and window treatments to items and images.

Create tenderness for yourself and your loved ones, find it easier to express appreciation and tenderness, and be more open to receive tender attention from others. This is the most feminine or yin of all the enhancements and is governed by the element Earth bringing essence of care, warmth, love and relationship. Place symbols of tenderness.

In your lounge room place a six-rod hollow metal wind chime. Wind chimes attract good chi. Ensure that it is a six-rod hollow metal wind chime. This wind chime is the best moving metal activator because it removes the density of the earth by attracting the energy of the earth in its hollow tubes. Change any angles or sharp edges of furniture, columns, shelves, pointed plants, ornaments, or objects to point away from where you and your loved ones sit. Hang crystals at large windows to reflect sunlight and create rainbows.

In your child's bedroom hang images of dragonflies or butterflies. Do not place tigers or lions, they represent predators nor negative messages such as 'Keep Out', this will influence your tender relationship with your child as well as harmony in the whole home.

Feng Shui practice also means creating tenderness in the gifts you give your loved ones. Give personalized gifts with your heart. Place your gift in soft tissue paper. Do not give clocks or watches these symbolise that you do not have time for them or that time is running out.

BALANCE and HARMONY

Feng Shui is an art and science of principles derived from ancient Eastern practices that is designed to balance and harmonise the home or workplace which in turn creates balance and harmony within oneself. If one's home is healthy, then the individual can be healthy. This also assists with better insight to make the right decision, especially when you are torn between opposing situations, ideas, or people as well as help in resolving conflicts between people or to keep conflicts from escalating. When balance or yin and yang is achieved in the environment a positive energy flow is created. There are many factors in an environment that can block this positive flow of energy, and one aspect is organisation.

Yin and yang are defined as two halves that together complete wholeness. When something is split or incomplete, it upsets the equilibrium of wholeness. This starts both halves chasing after each other as they seek a new balance with each other. Yang means "sunny or bright", and corresponds to the day and more active functions. Whereas yin, means "shady or dark", and corresponds to night and less active functions. These opposites are polarity required for harmonic balance. Opposing or contrary forces are complementary, interconnected, and interdependent in the natural world, and how they give rise to each other as they interrelate to one another. Duality exists in everything whether tangible or intangible, some examples are hot/cold, tall/short, or male/female. Duality is found in all and are parts of Oneness

Activate your Home or Office For in Health

Yang energy: white, heaven, male, active, day, sun, contraction, mountains, light colours, loud music, round shapes and round people, optimistic, energetic, young, outside and active.

Yin energy: black, earth, female, receptive, night, moon, expansion, valley, dark colours, silence or soft music, long shapes and tall people, pessimistic, exhausted, old, inside and passive.

When your life is out of balance, analyse the balance in your home and workplace. Balance the Five Elements: fire, water, wood, earth and metal. Also add air to the spaces. Each of these elements works independently and collectively to restore calm and bring energy to your space. Balance and harmony is imperative in Feng Shui practice, it is recommended that a Feng Shui Consultant is appointed to ensure this is created to its optimum level. However, below is a starter.

Earth – Earthy colour tones. Crystals or clay.
Metal – Silver or gold
Water – Blues. Water or glass.
Wood – Greens or browns. Timbers or plants.
Fire – Fiery colour tones. Sun or candles.

Create harmony for a stronger connection between who you are and what you do, to increase peace and harmony in your life as well as reduce the conflict, drama, and stress in your home or workplace. Create this in your landscape, home and workplace. To do this the five elements – wood, fire, earth, metal, and water – must be in harmony in each room/space.

When an element is not represented in an area, place something of that element. For instance, missing the wood element, place something to represent wood. When an element is overpowering, weaken it with the appropriate element from the weakening cycle. For example, an overpowering timber room, place fire elements such as reds or candles in the space for balance. When one element creates a lot of chaos, clash, or disaster, repaint the room.

Use the elements listed below in various combinations, enhance, weaken, or control your spaces. Ensure all of the elements are represented in each space.

Productive Cycle:
WOOD fuels FIRE
FIRE creates EARTH
EARTH produces METAL

METAL condenses or holds WATER
WATER feeds WOOD

Weakening Cycle:
WOOD reduces WATER
WATER reduces METAL
METAL reduces EARTH
EARTH reduces FIRE
FIRE reduces WOOD

Destructive Cycle:
WOOD consumes EARTH
EARTH dams WATER
WATER extinguishes FIRE
FIRE melts METAL
METAL cuts WOOD

Wood harnesses the power of creativity and expansion. Wood also represents birth, strength, flexibility and intuition. There must be proper balance in the use of wood in your space as too much creates overwhelment, stubbornness and inflexibility. Not enough wood creates lack of creativity, indecision and depression. Place plants, paper, furniture or textiles. .

Fire increases enthusiasm and leadership skill. In the home fire is used to encourage expressiveness, inspiration and boldness. With fire a perfect balance is essential. Too much fire creates anger, aggression, irritability and impulsive behaviour. A lack of fire creates emotional coldness, lack of vision, inexpressiveness and low self-esteem. Place some candles, electronics or natural sunlight.

Earth affects our physical strength. It creates grounding, balance and stability. An overabundance of earth in a space, creates a sensation of boredom, sluggishness and seriousness. Too little earth creates disorganisation, chaos and lack of focus. Place images of landscapes or square shapes. Do not place images such as snowy mountains.

Metal affects mental clarity and logic. It creates organisation, focus, righteousness and analytical abilities. Too much metal creates chattiness, overly critical thoughts and speaking without thinking. Too little metal creates cautiousness and lack of focus. Place items of iron, aluminium, gold or silver;

Water responds to spirituality and emotion. A balance of water creates inspiration, wisdom and insightfulness. Too much creates feelings of unbalanced growth and the sense of emotionally drowning. It can make you feel overwhelmed and overly social. Too little water creates lack of sympathy, loneliness, isolation, and stress. Try incorporating water into your space by adding blacks, blues or reflective surfaces.

FOCUS

When focus is in balance you have fewer distractions and stronger concentration, stay focused on your goals, it improves your motivation for finishing projects you start and helps to recover from conditions or circumstances that diminish your focus.

To maintain focus decluttering all your spaces in the home, workplace and yard is imperative. Everything must have its place and there must be order. Even when items are in a cupboard or drawers, it must be easily accessible and not jammed full of things that fall out or must be removed to get to other layers.

In business, always declutter desk and workplace before end the day. Return everything to its best Feng Shui position. Arrange the surface of your desk with Feng Shui principles. The nine directions or bagua is a map that can be applied to your desktop as well as your computer, just as it would be applied to the floor plan of a home or office. Different areas of the bagua are associated with different areas of your life, for health place as follows:

- The center of the desk represents health, do not have any clutter here. Place a yellow item or colour here.
- The right side of the center of the desk represents creativity and focus. Place silver, gold, or white colour here. Also place inspirational materials, such as quotes or books.
-The front right corner represents helpers and travel. Place a grey item or colour here including your address book, a travel guide or an image of a holiday location.
- For the computer place icons such as your health programs, or a folder containing pdfs/eBooks on wellness in the east of the screen which is the middle left hand side of the computer screen to enhance your health flow. For Personal fortune relationships, this can be established through a Personal Feng Shui analysis by a Feng Shui consultant.
-

For those who have a home office or work from home, you can apply the same Feng Shui principles as in any other work environment. Keep the entrance of your home neat, clean, and free of clutter, including the entrance to your office space. Even if clients do not attend this workplace this is essential in opening the flow of energy and welcoming positive improvements to your work life.

A variety of influences such as architecture, furniture, plumbing, colours, shapes, objects, symbols, landscape, and surrounding environment can lead to an inability to focus. Below are features and factors in your home or workplace that can interfere with focus, and what can be done to activate greater focus right away.

Bed Position
When bed is located on the same wall as the door, you cannot see the people coming into the room. Move bed. If moving the bed is not possible, hang a small mirror opposite the door so you can see anyone entering the bedroom. Do not sleep under a window. Moonlight on the head, brings trouble focusing during the daytime. If bed cannot be moved away from window. Place a heavy screen between your bed and the window.
For focus in the morning, remove electrical fields that interfere with focus during the night. Place alarm clocks at least 5 or 6 feet away from body unless they run on batteries.

Do not have a mirror reflecting the bed. A mirror that reflects your image when you are in bed scatters thoughts and create negative dreams. It also doubles health issues. This applies to any reflective surface such as a television screen. Move all mirrors and reflective surfaces so you cannot see your image in bed or cover them before going to bed.

Bathrooms near bedrooms create focus problems. Keep the bathroom door closed day and night. Do not place bed against a bathroom wall. If your bed must be against a bathroom wall, place a mirror behind the headboard facing the bathroom to deflect the flushing of your energy field.

Poison Arrows
Any architectural features, furniture and pointed objects that aim toward you are considered poison arrows. For example, corners of tables, desks or any comer of two walls that are in line with where you work or sleep.

A poison arrow directed at your body as you work will interrupt your focus. If you notice poison arrows where you sit or sleep from cabinets or bookcases place fabric or an item to cover the arrow. Ensure that all books on shelves, even shelves with doors, are flush with the edge of the shelf. This prevents shelves from creating a horizontal cutting energy that disturbs focus.

COMPASSION

Create a gentle ease of love and support in the way you relate to yourself and others. *"Be gentle first with yourself if you wish to be gentle with others." ~Lama Yeshe.*

- When we feel compassion for others, we feel kindness toward them, empathy, and a desire to help. It's the same when you are compassionate toward yourself. Self-compassion creates a caring space within you that is free of judgment. An important part of living a happy and fulfilling life includes being part of sharing, helping and supporting people you care about. It also includes being kind to strangers, and learning to replace envy and anger with understanding and empathy. Allow yourself to see that *everything* around you is sacred.

Enhance compassion in the southwest direction of your lounge room or bedroom by placing an image or statue of your 'Mother of Compassion': Kuan Yin, Mother Mary, Tara, Mother Theresa, Isis or someone who represents compassion to you.

-Feel more compassion for yourself, others, and for the world you live in

- Go easy on yourself when you try new things or make mistakes

- Show trust in others and treat them with patience and gentleness

- Have patience to listen to your inner voice and the advice of others
- Be more open to others

EMPOWERMENT/SELF-EMPOWERMENT

Manifest Your Power by being open to transform your life. When you start to change things, make the changes with the right attitude. Proceed fearlessly. Do not complain about the changes you need to make or it will block the ease of making them. Look for support available to you and believe you will have all the help you need. Let go of things and situations with joy. When something does not serve you anymore, be thankful for what you received from it. Recycle it to bless someone else. Place ornaments and move furniture with a sense of blessing. In between every change, take time to experience the impact and enjoy the process.

--Forgive yourself and release the past. Write a list of what you forgive yourself for or say it out aloud.

-Have courage to make necessary changes

-Create collaboration with all of the support available to you

-Love yourself and release judgment. Hold the intention that it will empower you to do your Feng Shui decluttering, cleaning, and activations now.

- Be more outgoing

- Learn how and when to say no. This is a crucial step towards reclaiming your personal sense of empowerment. You control your own choices.

ENHANCE YOUR CONNECTION TO HEAVEN

The direction connected to the Northwest is called Helpful People and Blessings or Connection to Heaven and help from Heaven, it also relates to patriarch and patronage luck representing the full force of Yang energy. This direction within the home or workspace aligns your connection with the outside world including your mentors, work colleagues, friends, networking, benefactors and business prospects.

Place an activation here for the energy to help attract beneficial people in your life. We all need somebody to help us. We all need a mentor. Mentors do not only refer to people who are in power who can teach us things or help us in achieving our goals, this also refers to people who may not be our senior in stature, age, experience, but are around us can is able to contribute to our success. Place silver bells and a singing bowl in this direction. Avoid water images as they will deplete the favourable energy.

In Feng Shui, by activating our Mentor's Luck we start to attract people who help us along the way. Begin by being positive yourself this starts the flow of a powerful positive aura, which in turn will attract people who are also positive.

This direction also supports the energy of travel, if you would like to travel more, express this energy here. Travel is also beneficial to health, new environments equals a new flow of Qi. Place travel photos, and maps. Photos of people who have helped you grow in life are also good to display or spiritual mentors, symbols, teachers, and angels that support us. Do not put a fire element, candles in the Northwest of home, lounge room, or other important rooms because it symbolizes fire at heaven's gate. If you have a fireplace in the Northwest, place a bowl of still water next to it, the water element represents diminishing the fire energy.

YOUR SENSES

Eyes- Use the combinations of red and gold or purple and silver to attract more passion. Do not limit when decorating with art. Displaying images of only one type, such as flowers or children, shows you are passionate about that subject only. Hang images representing good health, happiness and anything else you would like to show passion for. Never hang what you are passionate about in the bathroom.

Ears - Use water fountains or wind chimes that sound harmonious. Play background music the whole day. Open windows and listen to the wind and birds. Play soothing background sounds of ocean waves or nature.

Mouth- Have fruit in a bowl and Images of fruit. Ensure your refrigerator is at least half full of good food and tasty drinks. Also make your dining table luxurious with colourful plates, napkins and beautiful glasses.

Skin and sense of touch - Maintain the right body temperature. Circulate fresh air by opening the window or running a fan. Enjoy the touch of the right fabrics or materials on skin. Appoint a Feng Shui consultant to establish your personal elements, this way you can wear the ideal fabrics and colours for your personal Health direction that recharge you and works for you.

Sense of smell - The smell at any entrance should be positive and uplifting. Get rid of dusty and musty smells. Use refreshing essential oils, air filters, negative ion systems, incense, or lavender bags in closets/dense areas.

Quick tips

Connect to your space personally to empower your life. Display your favourite art or patterns you love to help forge a strong bond between you and your environment.

In order to make a room look and feel magnificent, you must think about adding gravity and balance to the space. Think about your home or workspace as a living, breathing entity that wants to feel the same. A bare dining or coffee table with art on the walls feels very different to a table that has a centrepiece displayed. This centrepiece creates visual focus that organizes the room in a new way, helping it to appear more settled.

Open space welcomes new opportunities and open space gives wellness and relationships room to flourish

and thrive. Clear space for happy conversations. By removing non-essential excess, it allows the flow for comfort and nestled joy.

Open your windows wide and often, and replace recycled air with a fresh Qi.

Activate your Home or Office For in Health

Invite guests over and feed them this indicates you are abundant enough to feed many mouths, you generate a prosperous energy and like energy attracts more like energy. This also enhances happiness in your space.

Appreciate the true abundance in your relationships and space. When you practice appreciation in your environment all those who come into your space feel love. When we notice and show gratitude for what is good in our life, it amplifies a trail for more success to our life.

Change your home or workspace by giving it beauty and order, and it will fill with purpose and clarity. Life imitates our environments, show and act with love daily and the big things you desire manifest more easily. When positive experiences occur around you, give thanks. This is a sign that more good things are on their way.

Life is divided into nine fields: prosperity, fame and reputation, relationships and love, creativity and children, skills and wisdom, helpful people and travel, career, family, and health. Analyse Your Qi Flow and Determine which areas in your life need the most work and a greater flow.

Keep things clean and organised.

When someone compliment you, thank them and let them know how happy it makes you.

Go out dancing and celebrate.

In your relationships, your task is to create harmony in your family, wherever they are.

Be spontaneous and creative.

Take enough time to enjoy people.

To have a great relationship with yourself, take a meditation class or listen to a guided meditation.

Be mindful of your boundaries. Help and mentor people but ensure you have boundaries, without them you will lose yourself in the relationship.

See your health and relationships as your greatest wealth and abundance.

Activate your Home or Office For in Health

Build strong bonds with your loved ones and colleagues.

To avoid games and drama in your life, avoid any kind of games, such as video games or board games, in the east and southwest of your home.

In the east direction of your home and workspace place objects made from wood, floral prints in wall papers and fabrics, pictures that are symbolic of vibrant good health. Personal artwork or items that represent what it is you desire to bring into your life in terms of health. Art improves the energy of both home and workspace. Ensure the art you select fits the needs of the room. For example; a bedroom or bathroom should have artwork that is sensual and soothing. Family rooms and workspaces are enhanced with art that energises; filled with bright, vibrant colours and images. The tone of the art must fit the tone of the room.

Vision boards and collages you make are the most powerful. Make it personal and put your own positive Qi into creating it.

If you are working with weight issues, find pictures representing your ideal body type.

Treat your body with respect and give it the energy of beauty and joy - it will inevitably attract good health and well-being.

The presence of Buddha creates instant tranquillity. Place a figure or image of Buddha in your home. Aroma therapy is another calming Feng shui practice. The daily use of essential oils will help purify, relax, and energise you and your environment.

Bamboo is considered to be a symbol of good luck and is thought to teach ultimate wisdom also it allows the spirit to flow freely and heal your being.

To ensure the flow of Qi does not rush upstairs or down, place a plant or another focal point at the side of the staircase or close off the stairs with a door or screen. Avoid bright red.

Do not leave wastebaskets, clutter, or dirt in any direction that you activate.

Activate General Directions, in lounge room, workspace and bedrooms unless otherwise stated – pertaining the connected direction.

Do not place dried flowers, the positive Qi no longer exists in these.

Many have discovered the benefits of Feng Shui. If you would like to invite more wellness in your life, begin with these principles and expand the energy in your home or workspace. In the eastern culture, those who find success through Feng Shui practices do not sell their homes once they become millionaires. They keep it for luck and continued good energy, even if they move into a new house.

Everything we do is controlled by the energy we put into it. Feng Shui helps release stagnated energy and escorts in good energy. Those who find the right balance in their homes discover that when the right energy is in place their success increases. Feng Shui is an ancient science and art that many people have had success with, and it's possible for you to have that same success, as well

For complete and comprehensive balancing, activations and cures for your home or workspace, contact a Feng Shui Consultant. Please note: Direction identification with a compass is the only way to get an accurate reading of your environment. More than half of the people who conduct their own Feng Shui compass readings do it incorrectly. It's imperative that it's accurate; creating analyses based on inaccurate readings is worse than doing nothing to correct or remedy inauspicious elements in your home.

Create a Vision board

A vision board is a paper or board where you put in the centre a recent image of yourself in a enhancing outfit, depending on the type of health you desire, ensure the image reflects this and what it means to you. Place images around it that represent vitality, wellness, images that make you happy, and images that represent your intentions, for example. You want to eat healthier, place fresh fruit, images of healthy skin or words that reflect this. Place your vision board in the East direction in your workspace or lounge room.

Chinese Proverb
*"When the heart is at ease, the body is **healthy**".*

Being Gracious and Appreciation

Being Gracious and feeling appreciation are powerful processes, and both invite a tremendous flow of positive Qi that continues to amplify as this is practised daily. The next pages are simple lists of statements and things that help us feel good. Use these lists, choose your favourites, rewrite them, add to them, and play with them. Make this a daily occupation. Feel good now! And your abundance for health, success, relationships and growth will come swiftly.

99 Things You Can Be Gracious for on Any Given Day
I am gracious for...

1) Blazing orange and magenta sunsets
2) Quiet dawns in the darkness of early morning
3) Jacaranda trees
4) Exotic flowers like lilies and orchids
5) Books
6) Comfy, warm home on a cold day
7) Neon-green newborn grass emerging in spring
8) Supportive, loyal friends

9) Giving and receiving
10) Art in all its forms
11) Sparkles on the surface of water
12) Sturdy strong trees
13) Strong bodies that move us
14) Fairy lights
15) The first spring flower rising up
16) Optimism
17) Positivity
18) Silliness
19) Gratitude!
20) Indoor plumbing
21) Laughing till your tummy hurts
22) Deep emotion and passion
23) Our guides and angels
24) Turquoise
25) Walks in nature
26) A favorite song
27) Dancing madly
28) The golden light on nearby mountains
29) Doors for privacy
30) Quantum physics
31) Infinity
32) Worlds upon worlds

33) Feng Shui
34) A warm soup in winter
35) Clear deep rushing rivers
36) Jumpers and jackets
37) Baby lambs, puppies, kittens
38) Food glorious food
39) Too many bubbles in a bubble bath
40) My skin
41) Goofy faces
42) My happy family
43) Technology that connects the world
44) Pen and paper
45) Renoir, Picasso, Van Gogh
46) Pungent fragrances of lavender, rosemary, mint, rose
47) Pop Music to rock out to
48) Wisdom through the ages
49) Words like wonderful, luscious and nourish
50) Mother Teresa
51) Modern day mystics
52) Playtime especially when we are all grown up
53) Looking at the night sky
54) Comfortable bed
55) Unfurling of a fern frond
56) Water! Drinking it and knowing we are mostly made of it

57) The universal language of music
58) Yellow
59) Scurrying possums
60) The bustle and mix of animals, people, cars and bikes in Melbourne
61) Stretching our bodies
62) Hugs and kisses
63) Sharing with like-minded friends
64) The whole intricate, multi-layered systems of our bodies
65) Siblings through thick and thin
66) Loving, caring, nurturing mothers
67) Steady, sensible, hardworking fathers
68) Double rainbows
69) The wonder of birth!
70) Peace, quiet, serenity
71) Cars that transport us
72) The internet
73) The brilliant, bright extravaganza of summer
74) The vast ocean – the waves and tides and immensity
75) The magic of life
76) Scientists and mathematicians
77) Magenta
78) Routines we can count on
79) The fact that our world is spinning and we feel stable

80) Tropical islands
81) Dancing and laughing
82) Red
83) Melodious singers
84) The beat of drums
85) Enjoying a cool salad on a hot summer day
86) Honesty and forthrightness – people you can count on
87) Exquisite rain falling
88) Blue, and all the myriad of shades of it
89) Eyes that are a window to the soul
90) Smiles
91) Love – agape love, family love, self-love
92) The feeling of joy that upwells from within
93) The Earth's incredible beauty
94) Purple
95) Other life in the universe that is undoubtedly there
96) Particles and waves dancing and disappearing
97) Confidence and Trust
98) Kind deeds and compassion
99) All the things left off this list…

Activate your Home or Office For in Health

NATURAL JOYS

Think about these one at a time before going on to the next one.

1. Being in love.
2. Laughing so hard your face hurts.
3. A hot shower.
4. No queues at the supermarket.
5. Taking a drive on a pretty road.
6. Hearing your favourite song on the radio.
7. Lying in bed listening to the rain outside.
8. Hot towels fresh out of the dryer.
9. Chocolate milkshake ... or vanilla ... or strawberry!
10. A bubble bath.
11. Giggling.
12. A good conversation.
13. Finding a note in your jacket from last winter.
14. Running through sprinklers.
15. Laughing for absolutely no reason at all.
16. Having someone tell you that you're beautiful.
17. Accidentally overhearing someone say something nice about you.
18. Waking up and realising you still have a few hours left to sleep.
19. Making new friends or spending time with old ones.

20. Having someone play with your hair.

21. Sweet dreams.

22. Making eye contact with a cute stranger.

23. Holding hands with someone you care about.

24. Running into an old friend and realising that some things (good or bad) never change.

25. Watching the expression on someone's face as they open a much-desired present from you.

26. Getting out of bed every morning and being grateful for another beautiful day.

27. Knowing that somebody misses you.

28. Getting a hug from someone you care about deeply.

29. Knowing you've done the right thing, no matter what other people think.

For more information about this author

And other books:

www.terminaashton.com

www.terminafengshui.com

www.perpelflame.com

www.thehappymagnet.com

www.ingramcontent.com/pod-product-compliance
Lightning Source LLC
Chambersburg PA
CBHW050442010526
44118CB00013B/1639